Non communicable diseases

Challenges involving non communicable diseases and how to overcome it

Marion drive

Table of contents

Chapter 1
What are non-communicable diseases
and their types?

Noncommunicable diseases (NCDs),
including heart disease, stroke, cancer,
diabetes, and chronic lung disease, are
collectively responsible for almost 70% of
all deaths worldwide. Almost
three-quarters of all NCD deaths, and
82% of the 16 million people who died
prematurely, or before reaching 70 years
of age, occur in low- and middle-income
countries.

The rise of NCDs has been driven by
primarily four major risk factors: tobacco
use, physical inactivity, the harmful use
of alcohol, and unhealthy diets.

The epidemic of NCDs poses
devastating health consequences for
individuals, families, and communities,
and threatens to overwhelm health
systems. The socioeconomic costs
associated with NCDs make the
prevention and control of these diseases
a major development imperative for the
21st century.
WHO's mission is to provide leadership
and the evidence base for international
action on surveillance, prevention, and
control of NCDs. Urgent government
action is needed to meet global targets to
reduce the burden of NCDs

Noncommunicable diseases (NCDs) kill
41 million people each year, equivalent to
71% of all deaths globally.
Each year, more than 15 million people
die from an NCD between the ages of 30
and 69 years; 85% of these "premature"

deaths occur in low- and middle-income countries.

77% of all NCD deaths are in low- and middle-income countries.

Cardiovascular diseases account for most NCD deaths, or 17.9 million people annually, followed by cancers (9.3 million), respiratory diseases (4.1 million), and diabetes (1.5 million).

These four groups of diseases account for over 80% of all premature NCD deaths.

Tobacco use, physical inactivity, the harmful use of alcohol, and unhealthy diets all increase the risk of dying from an NCD.

Detection, screening, and treatment of NCDs, as well as palliative care, are key components of the response to NCDs.

Mental Health Disorders

Mental, neurological, and substance use disorders are common in all regions of the world, affecting every community and age group across all income countries. While 14% of the global burden of disease is attributed to these disorders, most of the people affected – 75% in many low-income countries – do not have access to the treatment they need.

The WHO Mental Health Gap Action Program (mhGAP) aims at scaling up mental health services, especially for low- and middle-income countries. The program asserts that with proper care, psychosocial assistance and medication, tens of millions could be treated for depression, schizophrenia, and epilepsy, prevented from suicide, and begin to lead normal lives – even where resources are scarce.

Jan Swasthya Sahyog, (People's Health Support Group) is a nonprofit community health organization in central Chhattisgarh, India that treats thousands of tribal people each year with support from donors and grants from institutions like the Sir Ratan Tata Trust. Tribal people, India's indigenous citizens who often lived off the grid and have only recently been pushed into mainstream culture, makeup 38% of the population in Chhattisgarh.

A 2015 NPR report, "Why A Snakebite Victim In An Indian Village Won't Walk Through A Door" covered Manju Thakur, a community health worker with Jan Swasthya Sahyog. Originally from a nearby village, Thakur spoke to a support group of 20 psychiatric patients suffering from bipolar disorder, schizophrenia, and depression as well as others who came to work on anger management. Most patients in Bhamni, one of the larger villages in Achanakmar, blame their behavior on the supernatural – a common belief in a culture that widely accepts spirits in both humans and nature.

Raymond tells them the mind is like the body – it needs to be maintained and treated. Thakur says she has to be very convincing and sensitive to steer patients away from traditional healers, who perform rituals or prescribe herbs. She visits homes frequently and shares stories of other people who have recovered in hopes they will consider another type of treatment.
"[The village healer] said there's a ghost or spirit in me," says Chotilal Gond, a 30-year-old construction worker who has been hearing voices in his head. Gond had visited the tribal healer before a

community worker identified his issue and referred him to the clinic, where Thakur diagnosed him with schizophrenia and convinced him to take the drug olanzapine. Now, he comes to the monthly meetings she holds in the village.

Heart Attack
A heart attack happens when something blocks the blood flow to your heart so it can't get the oxygen it needs.
More than a million Americans have heart attacks each year. Heart attacks are also called myocardial infarctions (MI). "Myo" means muscle, cardiac refers to the heart, and "infarction" means the death of tissue because of a lack of blood supply. This tissue death can cause lasting damage to your heart muscle.

Cancer
is a disease in which some of the body's
cells grow uncontrollably and spread to
other parts of the body.
Cancer can start almost anywhere in the
human body, which is made up of trillions
of cells. Normally, human cells grow and
multiply (through a process called cell
division) to form new cells as the body
needs them. When cells grow old or
become damaged, they die, and new
cells take their place.
Sometimes this orderly process breaks
down, and abnormal or damaged cells
grow and multiply when they shouldn't.
These cells may form tumors, which are
lumps of tissue. Tumors can be
cancerous or not cancerous (benign).

Cancerous tumors spread into, or invade
nearby tissues and can travel to distant
places in the body to form new tumors (a

process called metastasis). Cancerous tumors may also be called malignant tumors. Many cancers form solid tumors, but cancers of the blood, such as leukemias, generally do not.
Benign tumors do not spread into, or invade nearby tissues. When removed, benign tumors usually don't grow back, whereas cancerous tumors sometimes do. Benign tumors can sometimes be quite large, however. Some can cause serious symptoms or be life-threatening,

Diff between cancer cells and normal cells
Cancer cells differ from normal cells in many ways. For instance, cancer cells: grow in the absence of signals telling them to grow. Normal cells only grow when they receive such signals.

ignore signals that normally tell cells to stop dividing or to die (a process known as programmed cell death, or apoptosis).

invade into nearby areas and spread to other areas of the body. Normal cells stop growing when they encounter other cells, and most normal cells do not move around the body.

tell blood vessels to grow toward tumors. These blood vessels supply tumors with oxygen and nutrients and remove waste products from tumors.

hide from the immune system. The immune system normally eliminates damaged or abnormal cells.

trick the immune system into helping cancer cells stay alive and grow. For instance, some cancer cells convince immune cells to protect the tumor instead of attacking it.

accumulate multiple changes in their chromosomes, such as duplications and

deletions of chromosome parts. Some cancer cells have double the normal number of chromosomes.
rely on different kinds of nutrients than normal cells. In addition, some cancer cells make energy from nutrients in a different way than most normal cells. This lets cancer cells grow more quickly. Many times, cancer cells rely so heavily on these abnormal behaviors that they can't survive without them. Researchers have taken advantage of this fact, developing therapies that target the abnormal features of cancer cells. For example, some cancer therapies prevent blood vessels from growing toward tumors, essentially starving the tumor of needed nutrients.

How does cancer develop
Cancer is caused by certain changes to genes, the basic physical units of

inheritance. Genes are arranged in long strands of tightly packed DNA called chromosomes.

Cancer is a genetic disease—that is, it is caused by changes to genes that control the way our cells function, especially how they grow and divide.

Genetic changes that cause cancer can happen because of errors that occur as cells divide.

of damage to DNA caused by harmful substances in the environment, such as the chemicals in tobacco smoke and ultraviolet rays from the sun. (Our Cancer Causes and Prevention section has more information.)

they were inherited from our parents.

The body normally eliminates cells with damaged DNA before they turn cancerous. But the body's ability to do so goes down as we age. This is part of the reason why there is a higher risk of cancer later in life.

Each person's cancer has a unique combination of genetic changes. As cancer continues to grow, additional changes will occur. Even within the same tumor, different cells may have different genetic changes.

Types of genes that cause cancer

The genetic changes that contribute to cancer tend to affect three main types of genes—proto-oncogenes, tumor suppressor genes, and DNA repair genes. These changes are sometimes called "drivers" of cancer.

Proto-oncogenes are involved in normal cell growth and division. However, when these genes are altered in certain ways or are more active than normal, they may become cancer-causing genes (or oncogenes), allowing cells to grow and survive when they should not.

Tumor suppressor genes are also involved in controlling cell growth and division. Cells with certain alterations in tumor suppressor genes may divide in an uncontrolled manner.

DNA repair genes are involved in fixing damaged DNA. Cells with mutations in these genes tend to develop additional mutations in other genes and changes in their chromosomes, such as duplications and deletions of chromosome parts. Together, these mutations may cause the cells to become cancerous.

As scientists have learned more about the molecular changes that lead to cancer, they have found that certain mutations commonly occur in many types of cancer. Now there are many cancer treatments available that target gene mutations found in cancer. A few of these treatments can be used by anyone with cancer that has the targeted mutation, no matter where cancer started growing

When cancer spreads
In metastasis, cancer cells break away from where they first formed and form new tumors in other parts of the body. Cancer that has spread from the place where it first formed to another place in the body is called metastatic cancer. The process by which cancer cells spread to other parts of the body is called metastasis.

Metastatic cancer has the same name and the same type of cancer cells as the original, or primary, cancer. For example, breast cancer that forms a metastatic tumor in the lung is metastatic, not lung cancer.

Under a microscope, metastatic cancer cells generally look the same as cells of original cancer. Moreover, metastatic cancer cells and cells of original cancer usually have some molecular features in common, such as the presence of specific chromosome changes.

In some cases, treatment may help prolong the lives of people with metastatic cancer. In other cases, the primary goal of treatment for metastatic cancer is to control the growth of cancer or to relieve the symptoms it is causing. Metastatic tumors can cause severe damage to how the body functions, and most people who die of cancer die of metastatic disease.

Tissue changes that are not cancer

Not every change in the body's tissues is cancer. Some tissue changes may develop into cancer if they are not treated, however. Here are some examples of tissue changes that are not cancer but, in some cases, are monitored because they could become cancer:

Hyperplasia occurs when cells within a tissue multiply faster than normal and extra cells build up. However, the cells and the way the tissue is organized still look normal under a microscope. Hyperplasia can be caused by several factors or conditions, including chronic irritation.

Dysplasia is a more advanced condition than hyperplasia. In dysplasia, there is also a buildup of extra cells. But the cells look abnormal and there are changes in how the tissue is organized. In general, the more abnormal the cells and tissue look, the greater the chance that cancer will form. Some types of dysplasia may need to be monitored or treated, but others do not. An example of dysplasia is an abnormal mole (called a dysplastic nevus) that forms on the skin. A dysplastic nevus can turn into melanoma, although most do not.

Carcinoma in situ is an even more advanced condition. Although it is sometimes called stage 0 cancer, it is not cancer because the abnormal cells do not invade nearby tissue the way that cancer cells do. But because some carcinomas in situ may become cancer, they are usually treated.

Normal cells may become cancer cells. Before cancer cells form in tissues of the body, the cells go through abnormal changes called hyperplasia and dysplasia. In hyperplasia, there is an increase in the number of cells in an organ or tissue that appear normal under a microscope. In dysplasia, the cells look abnormal under a microscope but are not cancer. Hyperplasia and dysplasia may or may not become cancer.

Types of cancer
There are more than 100 types of cancer. Types of cancer are usually named for the organs or tissues where the cancers form. For example, lung cancer starts in the lung, and brain cancer starts in the brain. Cancers also may be described by the type of cell that formed them, such as an epithelial cell or a squamous cell.
You can search NCI's website for information on specific types of cancer based on cancer's location in the body or by using our A to Z List of Cancers. We also have information on childhood cancers and cancers in adolescents and young adults.

Here are some categories of cancers that begin in specific types of cells:

Carcinoma
Carcinomas are the most common type of cancer. They are formed by epithelial cells, which are the cells that cover the inside and outside surfaces of the body. There are many types of epithelial cells, which often have a column-like shape when viewed under a microscope. Carcinomas that begin in different epithelial cell types have specific names:

Adenocarcinoma is cancer that forms in epithelial cells that produce fluids or mucus. Tissues with this type of epithelial cell are sometimes called glandular tissues. Most cancers of the breast, colon, and prostate are adenocarcinomas.

Basal cell carcinoma is cancer that begins in the lower or basal (base) layer of the epidermis, which is a person's outer layer of skin.

Squamous cell carcinoma is cancer that forms in squamous cells, which are epithelial cells that lie just beneath the outer surface of the skin. Squamous cells also line many other organs, including the stomach, intestines, lungs, bladder, and kidneys. Squamous cells look flat, like fish scales, when viewed under a microscope. Squamous cell carcinomas are sometimes called epidermoid carcinomas.

Transitional cell carcinoma is cancer that forms in a type of epithelial tissue called transitional epithelium, or urothelium. This tissue, which is made up of many layers of epithelial cells that can get

bigger and smaller, is found in the linings
of the bladder, ureters, part of the
kidneys (renal pelvis), and a few other
organs. Some cancers of the bladder,
ureters, and kidneys are transitional cell
carcinomas.

Sarcoma
Soft tissue sarcoma forms in soft tissues
of the body, including muscle, tendons,
fat, blood vessels, lymph vessels,
nerves, and tissue around joints.
Sarcomas are cancers that form in bone
and soft tissues, including muscle, fat,
blood vessels, lymph vessels, and

fibrous tissue (such as tendons and ligaments).

Osteosarcoma is the most common cancer of the bone. The most common types of soft tissue sarcoma are leiomyosarcoma, Kaposi sarcoma, malignant fibrous histiocytoma, liposarcoma, and dermatofibrosarcoma protuberans.

Leukemia
Cancers that begin in the blood-forming tissue of the bone marrow are called leukemias. These cancers do not form solid tumors. Instead, large numbers of abnormal white blood cells (leukemia cells and leukemic blast cells) build up in the blood and bone marrow, crowding out normal blood cells. The low level of normal blood cells can make it harder for

the body to get oxygen to its tissues, control bleeding, or fight infections. There are four common types of leukemia, which are grouped based on how quickly the disease gets worse (acute or chronic) and on the type of blood cell cancer starts in (lymphoblastic or myeloid). Acute forms of leukemia grow quickly and chronic forms grow more slowly.

Carcinogenesis is the process in which normal cells turn into cancer cells. Carcinogenesis is the series of steps that take place as a normal cell becomes a cancer cell. Cells are the smallest units of the body and they make up the body's tissues. Each cell contains genes that guide the way the body grows, develops, and repairs itself. Many genes control whether a cell lives or dies divides (multiplies), or takes on special functions,

such as becoming a nerve cell or a
muscle cell.

Changes (mutations) in genes occur
during carcinogenesis.
Changes (mutations) in genes can cause
normal controls in cells to break down.
When this happens, cells do not die
when they should and new cells are
produced when the body does not need
them. The buildup of extra cells may
cause a mass (tumor) to form.
Tumors can be benign or malignant
(cancerous). Malignant tumor cells
invade nearby tissues and spread to
other parts of the body. Benign tumor
cells do not invade nearby tissues or
spread.

A stroke, also known as a transient
ischemic attack or cerebrovascular
accident, happens when blood flow to the

brain is blocked. This prevents the brain from getting oxygen and nutrients from the blood. Without oxygen and nutrients, brain cells begin to die within minutes. Sudden bleeding in the brain can also cause a stroke if it damages brain cells.

A stroke is a medical emergency. A stroke can cause lasting brain damage, long-term disability, or even death. Signs of a stroke can range from mild weakness to paralysis or numbness on one side of the face or body. Other signs include a sudden and severe headache, sudden weakness, trouble seeing, and trouble speaking or understanding speech.
If you think you or someone else is having a stroke, call 9-1-1 right away. Do not drive to the hospital or let someone else drive you. Call an ambulance so that medical personnel can begin life-saving

treatment on the way to the emergency room. During a stroke, every minute counts.

At the hospital, a stroke team will assess your condition and treat your stroke with medicine, surgery, or another procedure. Your recovery will depend on how severe your stroke was and how quickly you got treatment. A rehabilitation plan may help you do the same things you used to do before your stroke.

Types of strokes. The most common type of stroke is ischemic stroke. This happens when plaque or a blood clot blocks blood flow to an artery in or on the brain. Hemorrhagic stroke is less common. This happens when a blood vessel breaks open and leaks blood into the brain. A transient ischemic attack (TIA) is similar to an ischemic stroke, but the blood clot breaks up after a short time, usually before there is long-term damage.

Diabetes

Type 2 Diabetes Mellitus is a chronic condition that is largely preventable and manageable but difficult to cure. Management concentrates on keeping blood sugar levels as close to normal ("euglycemia") as possible without presenting undue patient danger. This can usually be with close dietary management, exercise, and the use of appropriate medications (insulin only in the case of type 1 diabetes mellitus. Oral medications may be used in the case of type 2 diabetes, as well as insulin). Patient education, understanding, and participation are vital since the complications of diabetes are far less common and less severe in people who have well-managed blood sugar levels.

Wider health problems may accelerate the deleterious effects of diabetes. These include smoking, elevated cholesterol levels, obesity, high blood pressure, and lack of regular exercise

Although chronic kidney disease (CKD) is not currently identified as one of WHO's main targets for global NCD control, there is compelling evidence that CKD is not only common, harmful, and treatable but also a major contributing factor to the incidence and outcomes of at least three of the diseases targeted by WHO (diabetes, hypertension, and CVD).CKD strongly predisposes to hypertension and CVD; diabetes, hypertension, and CVD are all major causes of CKD; and major risk factors for diabetes, hypertension, and CVD (such as obesity and smoking) also cause or exacerbate CKD. In addition, among people with diabetes, hypertension, or CVD, the subset who also have CKD is at the highest risk of adverse outcomes and high health care costs. Thus, CKD, diabetes, and cardiovascular disease are closely associated conditions that often coexist; share common risk factors and treatments; and would benefit from a coordinated global approach to prevention and control.

Chronic Respiratory Diseases (CRDs) are diseases of the lungs and airways. According to the World Health Organization (WHO), hundreds of millions of people have CRDs.Common CRDs are Asthma, Chronic obstructive pulmonary disease, Occupational lung disease, and Pulmonary hypertension. While CRDs are not curable, various treatments are available to help improve the quality of life for individuals who have them. Most treatments involve dilating major airways to improve shortness of breath among other symptoms.The main risk factors for developing CRDs are tobacco smoking, indoor and outdoor air pollution, allergens, and occupational risks.

Chapter 2

Causes of non-communicable diseases

Ecological diseases
NCDs incorporate numerous ecological diseases covering a general class of avoidable and undeniable human medical issues brought about by outside factors, like daylight, nourishment, contamination, and way of life decisions.

The diseases of prosperity are non-irresistible diseases with natural causes. Models include:

Many kinds of cardiovascular infection (CVD)

Ongoing obstructive pneumonic infection (COPD) brought about by smoking tobacco

Diabetes mellitus type 2

Lower back torment brought about by too little activity

Unhealthiness brought about by too little food or eating some unacceptable sorts of food (for example scurvy from the absence of L-ascorbic acid)

Skin malignant growth brought about by radiation from the sun

Weight

Acquired illness

Hereditary problems are brought about by blunders in hereditary data that

produce diseases in the impacted individuals. The beginning of these hereditary blunders can be:
Unconstrained blunders or changes to the genome:
An adjustment of chromosome numbers, like Down disorder.
A deformity in quality is brought about by transformation, like Cystic fibrosis.
An expansion in how much hereditary data, like Chimerism or Heterochromia.
Cystic fibrosis is an illustration of an acquired sickness that is brought about by a change in quality. The flawed quality debilitates the ordinary development of sodium chloride all through cells, which causes the bodily fluid discharging organs to deliver strangely thick bodily fluid. The quality is latent, implying that an individual priority two duplicates of the flawed quality for them to foster the illness. Cystic fibrosis influences the

respiratory, stomach-related, and regenerative frameworks, as well as the perspiration organs. The bodily fluid discharged is exceptionally thick and blocks ways in the lungs and gastrointestinal systems. This bodily fluid causes issues with breathing and with the processing and ingestion of supplements.

Acquired hereditary mistakes from guardians:
Predominant hereditary diseases, like Huntington's, require the legacy of one incorrect quality to be communicated. Latent hereditary diseases require the legacy of mistaken qualities to be communicated and this is one explanation they cooperate.

Worldwide wellbeing

Passings from noncommunicable diseases per million people in 2012 Alluded to as a "way of life" infection, because most of these diseases are preventable sicknesses, the most widely recognized foundations for non-communicable diseases (NCD) incorporate tobacco use (smoking), risky liquor use, horrible eating routines (maximum usage of sugar, salt, soaked fats, and trans unsaturated fats) and actual dormancy. Right now, NCD kills 36 million individuals every year, a number that by certain evaluations is supposed to ascend by 17-24% within the following ten years.

By and large, numerous NCDs were related to the monetary turn of events and were purported as "diseases of the rich". The weight of non-communicable diseases in agricultural nations has expanded be that as it may, with an expected 80% of the four principal sorts of NCDs — cardiovascular diseases, malignant growths, persistent respiratory diseases, and diabetes — presently happening in low-and center pay nations. Activity Plan for the Worldwide Technique for the Counteraction and Control of non-communicable Diseases and with 66% of individuals who are impacted by diabetes presently dwelling in emerging countries, NCD can at this point not be viewed as only an issue influencing the well-off assessment of the financial effect of ongoing non-communicable diseases in chose nations. New WHO report: passings from non-communicable diseases are on the ascent, with creating world hit hardest. As recently expressed, in 2008 alone, NCDs were the reason for 63% of passings around the world; a number that is supposed to rise impressively sooner rather than later on the off chance that actions are not taken.

If current development patterns are kept up with, by 2020, NCDs will ascribe to 7 out of every 10 passings in non-industrial nations, killing 52 million individuals yearly overall by 2030. With measurements, for example, these, it shocks no one that global elements like the World Wellbeing Association and World Bank Human Advancement Organization have recognized the counteraction and control of NCDs as an inexorably significant conversation thing on the worldwide wellbeing plan.

Financial aspects
Beforehand, persistent NCDs were viewed as an issue restricted for the most part to big league salary nations, while irresistible diseases appeared to

influence low-pay nations. The weight of sickness credited to NCDs has been assessed at 85% in industrialized countries, 70% in center pay countries, and almost half in nations with the least public incomes. In 2008, ongoing NCDs represented over 60% (north of 35 million) of the 57 million passings around the world. Given the worldwide populace appropriation, practically 80% of passings due to constant NCDs overall currently happen in low and center pay nations, while just 20% happen in higher pay nations.

Public economies are experiencing huge misfortunes due to unexpected losses or powerlessness to work coming about because of coronary illness, stroke, and diabetes. For example, China is supposed to lose generally $558 billion in public pay somewhere in the range of 2005 and 2015 because of early passings. In 2005, coronary illness, stroke, and diabetes caused an expected misfortune in worldwide dollars of public pay of 9 billion in India and 3 billion in Brazil.

Non-appearance and presenteeism
The weight of persistent NCDs including psychological well-being conditions is felt in work environments all over the planet, outstandingly because of raised degrees of non-attendance, or nonappearance from work on account of ailment, and presenteeism, or efficiency lost from staff coming to work and performing beneath typical principles because of chronic weakness. For instance, the Unified Realm encountered a deficiency of around 175 million days in 2006 to the nonappearance of disease among a functioning populace of 37.7 million individuals. The assessed cost of

nonappearances because of disease was more than 20 billion pounds in a similar year. The cost because of presenteeism is probable significantly bigger, even though techniques for dissecting the financial effects of presenteeism are as yet being created. Techniques for dissecting the unmistakable working environment effects of NCDs versus different sorts of the medical issue are additionally as yet being created.

Tobacco is the main preventable reason of death on the planet and causes a few million passings every year around the world. Tobacco utilization influences each organ in the body and is a gamble factor for six of the eight driving reasons for passings on the planet.
Handed-down tobacco smoke is additionally perilous to wellbeing and

causes coronary illness and numerous serious respiratory and cardiovascular diseases in grown-ups, which can prompt passing. An expected 700 million kids, or close to half of the world's youngsters, inhale air contaminated by tobacco smoke, especially at home. There is no protected degree of openness to handing down tobacco smoke; just 100 percent without smoke conditions give viable insurance.

Despite negative social, monetary, and well-being impacts from the unsafe utilization of liquor, utilization of liquor stays a typical overall phenomenon. Changing degrees of utilization have to do with the monetary turn of events, social standards, accessibility of liquor, and liquor regulation. For instance, nations with higher pay for the most part polish off more liquor and have the most elevated measure of hard-core boozing episodes. Nonetheless, the outcomes of the unsafe utilization of liquor have searched the world. Liquor utilization added to practically 6% of all passings worldwide in 2012. This is because liquor is a huge causal element of noncommunicable diseases, for example, cardiovascular diseases and malignant growths notwithstanding liquor-related wounds including street car accidents and brutality (WHO, 2015).

Irresistible diseases can be brought about by:
Microscopic organisms. These one-cell living beings are answerable for ailments like strep throat, urinary parcel contaminations, and tuberculosis.
Infections. Significantly more modest than microscopic organisms, infections

cause a huge number of diseases going from the normal cold to Helps.
Parasites. Many skin diseases, like ringworm and competitor's foot, are brought about by parasites. Different sorts of growths can contaminate your lungs or sensory system.
Parasites. Intestinal sickness is brought about by a little parasite that is sent by a mosquito chomp. Different parasites might be communicated to people from creature excrement.
Direct contact
A simple method for getting the most irresistible diseases is by interacting with an individual or a creature with the contamination. Irresistible diseases can be spread through direct contact, for example,

One individual to the next. Irresistible diseases usually spread through the immediate exchange of microorganisms, infections, or different microbes starting with one individual and then onto the next. This can happen when a person with the bacterium or infection contacts, kisses, hacks, or wheezes on somebody who isn't infected. These microorganisms can likewise spread through the trading of body liquids from sexual contact. The individual who passes the microorganism might have no side effects of the illness, yet may essentially be a transporter.

Creature to individual. Being nibbled or scratched by a tainted creature — even a pet — can make you debilitated and, in outrageous conditions, can be lethal. Dealing with creature waste can be risky, as well. For instance, you can get toxoplasmosis disease by scooping your feline's litter box.

Mother to an unborn kid. A pregnant lady might pass microorganisms that make irresistible diseases to her unborn child. A few microorganisms can go through the placenta or bosom milk. Microorganisms in the vagina can likewise be communicated to the child during birth.

Aberrant contact

Sickness causing organic entities additionally can be passed by aberrant contact. Numerous microbes can wait on a lifeless thing, for example, a tabletop, door handle, or spigot handle.

At the point when you contact a door handle taken care of by somebody sick with influenza or a cold, for instance, you can get the microbes the person abandoned. If you, contact your eyes, mouth, or nose before cleaning up, you might become tainted.

Bug chomps
A few microbes depend on bug transporters — like mosquitoes, insects, lice, or ticks — to move from one host to another. These transporters are known as vectors. Mosquitoes can convey the intestinal sickness parasite or West Nile infection. Deer ticks might convey the bacteria

Chapter 3

Challenges involving noncommunicable diseases

Foundation challenges
As per studies, while political thoughtfulness regarding NCDs has expanded, in numerous nations there is as yet deficient thoughtfulness regarding this issue. For instance, as per a 2015 World Wellbeing Association overview of nations' ability, just 45% of nations

detailed having an NCD policy. In situations where there are framework strategies or projects, there are many times still serious financial plan problems. Infrastructure issues can be characterized into classifications including the absence of preventive foundation, limitations on admittance to medication, limitations on essential medical care, and limitations on admittance to innovation.

Monetary difficulties
Non-communicable diseases cause 35 million passings overall every year and are a significant snag to the improvement of countries. These diseases have seriously impacted poor people and weak individuals of the general public and are hauling them into the void of poverty. Dealing with these diseases is conceivable by controlling their gamble

factors and utilizing the encounters of different nations and the master exhortation of global associations. Then again, numerous items that increment NCDs are beneficial for organizations. As per studies, monetary difficulties can be isolated into benefit arranged, monetary precariousness, and fruitless execution of neediness decrease plans.

Segment difficulties
Movement enormously affects the example of life. The resident takes in the dirtied air and eats cheap food and his well-being is imperiled. Then again, the difference in the age pyramid has changed to the moderately aged populace. The populace maturing list in the nation has expanded from 14.8% to 39.5%. That is, for each 100 individuals younger than 15 in the country, around 40 older individuals live in Iran. 73.3% of

the older live in metropolitan regions and 26.7% in provincial areas. According to the review, segment difficulties can be ordered into the classes of maturing populace and relocation.

The executive's challenges Inappropriately or ineffectively overseeing metropolitan arranging conveys many dangers that affect NCD rate and mortality. For instance, it gets a critical increment in air contamination and inactive living. In 2012, roughly 75% of the total populace was presented to specific particles at focuses higher than those predetermined in World Wellbeing Association rules. In some big league salary nations, for example, Europe and North America, air contamination has declined in late a long time because of broad endeavors to diminish ozone-depleting substances and particulate matter. Management difficulties can be grouped by concentrating on the classes of quick and spontaneous metropolitan preparation, scurry in arranging, and absence of coordination inside and outside the area.

NCDs are many times described by interconnected circumstances and logical results chains. So distinguishing a particular element that prompts its decrease is extremely challenging and testing. Well-being advancement and infection counteraction are significant for NCDs that are related to various gamble factors that give a brilliant open door to mediation at the segment level. A large number of the gamble factors for NCDs are connected with the air we inhale, the food and drink we eat and drink, and the amount we move our bodies. In any case, overall to diminish non-communicable diseases, reinforce worldwide limits, lessen risk factors for NCDs and place social determinants by establishing wellbeing advancing conditions, reinforce wellbeing frameworks to carry out avoidance and control of NCDs, and Giving social determinants through individuals focused essential medical services can assume a powerful part.

Diets and Way of life
Before irresistible and parasitic diseases were the primary drivers of death, however, in the new many years, NCDs have supplanted them and have turned into the primary driver of passing. This might be credited to the difference in diet propensities and way of life throughout the long term, which can be delegated to a shift of illness designs in people. Different dietary elements, for example,

meat, entire grain items, sound dietary examples, sugar-improved drink utilization, and iron-based counts calories have an undeniable relationship with NCDs. Moreover, the maximum usage of handled meat and sugar-improved refreshments, joined with another unfortunate way of life factors, for example, a high weight file (BMI), actual idleness, and smoking have an undeniable relationship with NCDs. Entire grain items are free of the BMI and make defensive impacts, because of their high fiber items and capacity to gradually deliver glucose into flow; hence, this diminishes the postprandial insulin reaction and may further develop insulin awareness.

Dietary progress portrays the progressions underway, handling, accessibility, dietary utilization, and energy use. Further, the idea becomes more extensive and includes body arrangement, anthropometrical boundaries, and active work. The utilization of dietary progress terms emerges because of the shift to western weight control plans in agricultural nations specifically. Conventional food in many nations is better, normal, and more extravagant in fiber, and the cereal has been supplanted by undesirable handled food that is wealthy in sugars and fats, creature source food sources, and refined carbs. Thus, low and center-pay nations have seen quick changes in sustenance progress and fast expansions in NCDs. High food utilization and declining actual work rates happen all the while, bringing about NCDs. The primary element, owing to actual latency, is the fast and persistent advancement in innovation. The simple admittance to present-day innovation and assembling in houses and work environments, including machines, vehicles, and work saving innovation, make life more straightforward however unhealthier according to the viewpoint of lessening the gamble of NCDs

Chapter 4

Instructions to prevent non-communicable diseases

Handle and plan food securely
Food can convey microorganisms. Wash hands, utensils, and surfaces frequently while setting up any food, particularly crude meat. Continuously wash foods grown from the ground. Cook and keep food varieties at appropriate temperatures. Try not to forget about food - refrigerate expeditiously.

Wash hands frequently
One of the main sound propensities to forestall the spread of microbes is to clean your hands. Our hands can convey microbes, so it is vital to wash them frequently, regardless of whether they look messy.
When to Clean up
Make a point to clean your hands before and then afterward:
Utilizing the restroom or changing diapers

Eating
Preparing or serving food
Treating a cut or wound
Contact with a debilitated individual
Putting on and eliminating defensive gear
like a facial covering
Clean your hands after these activities:
Hacking, sniffling or cleaning out your
nose
Contacting someone else's hands or
contacting a creature or pet
Dealing with trash
Contacting as often as possible
contacted regions (door handles) or
polluted things (grimy clothing or dishes).
Step-by-step instructions to Wash Hands
with Cleanser and Water
Wet hands and apply cleanser.
Rub your hands for no less than 20
seconds. Scour all surfaces.
Wash hands.

Dry hands with a spotless material or paper towel. If in a public spot, utilize the paper towel to switch off the fixture.

Then, toss in the junk.

*While aiding a youngster, clean up first, and afterward your own.

Step-by-step instructions to Clean Hands with Hand Sanitizer

Use hand sanitizer on the off chance that cleanser and water are not accessible and on the off chance that your hands don't look grimy. To be viable, hand sanitizer should have something like 60% liquor content.

Apply hand sanitizer to two hands.

Rub hands covering all surfaces until dry. Assuming your hands dry before 10 seconds you didn't utilize enough. Apply more and rehash.

*Albeit not so successful as cleaning up with cleanser and water or utilizing hand

sanitizer, pre-saturated purifying towelettes with no less than 60% liquor content can be another option.

Clean and sanitize ordinarily utilized surfaces
Microorganisms can live on surfaces. Cleaning with cleanser and water is normally enough. In any case, you ought to clean your restroom and kitchen routinely. Sanitize different regions assuming somebody in the house is sick. You can utilize an EPA-guaranteed sanitizer (search for the EPA enrollment number on the name) or a detergent arrangement.

Hack and sniffle into a tissue or your sleeve
Assuming you are wiped out, the air that emerges from your mouth when you hack or sniffle might contain microbes.

Somebody nearby can take in your air, or contact a surface defiled with your microorganisms, and become sick. Hack or wheeze into a tissue or your shirt sleeve-not into your hands. Make sure to discard the tissue and clean it up. You can wear a facial covering when you are wiped out with a hack or sniffling sickness. Figure out how to put on and eliminate a facial covering.

Try not to share individual things
Try not to share individual things that can't be cleaned, similar as toothbrushes and razors, or dividing towels among washes. Needles ought to never be shared, ought to just be utilized once, and afterward discarded appropriately.

Get immunization
Immunizations can forestall numerous irresistible diseases. You ought to get a

few immunizations in youth, some as a grown-up, and some for extraordinary circumstances like pregnancy and travel. Ensure you and your family are state-of-the-art on your inoculations. If your normal specialist doesn't offer the antibody you want, visit the Grown-up Vaccination and Travel Facility.

Try not to contact wild creatures
You and your pets ought to try not to contact wild creatures which can convey microbes that cause irresistible diseases. On the off chance that you are chomped, converse with your PCP. Ensure that your pet's immunizations are cutting-edge.
Remain at home when debilitated
At the point when you are debilitated, remain at home and rest. You will recover sooner, and won't spread microorganisms.

www.ingramcontent.com/pod-product-compliance
Lightning Source LLC
Chambersburg PA
CBHW071446150726
48000CB00006B/2464